FRACKING AND HEALTH

facts vs. fiction

A publication of the

ACSH American Council on Science and Health
Science. Not Hype.

Written by
William Kucewiez

Based on a book authored by
Theodore F. Them, MD, MS, PhD, MPH, FACOEM

American Council on Science and Health
1995 Broadway, Suite 202
New York, New York 10023-5860
Tel. (212) 362-7044. Fax (212) 362-4919
URL: http://www.acsh.org. Email: acsh@acsh.org

Publisher Name: American Council on Science and Health
Title: Fracking and Health: Facts vs. Fiction
Price: $6.95
Author: William Kucewiez
Subject (general): Science and Health
Publication Year: 2014
Binding Type (i.e. perfect (soft) or hardcover): Perfect

ISBN: 978-0-9910055-2-9

ACKNOWLEDGEMENTS

This publication is based on the position paper *Hydraulic Fracturing in the Marcellus Shale: Water and Health, Facts vs. Fiction* (ISBN 978-0-9910055-1-2) authored by Dr. Theodore F. Them, and published by the American Council on Science and Health. The following people reviewed the original paper on which this summary is based:

JILL KRIESKY, PH.D.
Associate Director of the Southwest Pennsylvania Environmental Health Project
McMurray, PA

MICHAEL HOLLAND, MD, FACMY, FACOEM, FACEP
Toxicologist at Glen Falls Hospital
Glen Falls, NY

ANTHONY J. GRIPPO, MD, MPH
Associate Physician, Section of Occupational Medicine, Guthrie Clinic, Ltd.
Sayre, PA

ISAAC ORR
Research Fellow at The Heartland Institute
Chicago, IL

TABLE OF CONTENTS

E. Executive Summary....7

1. Introduction....9

2. U.S. Shale Gas Production....11

3. The Marcellus Shale....13

4. Recovery Technologies....17

5. Hydrofracturing and Human Health....21

6. Conclusions....23

7. References....25

EXECUTIVE SUMMARY

Shale gas is playing an increasingly important role in America's energy future. Half of all U.S. natural gas production is expected to come from shale by the year 2040. The most productive gas shales are organic rich "black" shales, such as the Devonian Marcellus Formation, or Marcellus Shale, a sedimentary rock formation deposited over 350 million years ago in a shallow inland sea located where the Appalachian Mountains in the eastern United States now stand.

The present-day revolution in shale gas took place virtually overnight. In the five years from 2004 to 2009, U.S. shale-gas production quadrupled. The advent of horizontal drilling and hydraulic fracturing have facilitated the expansion of modern shale-gas development. The technology involves drilling a vertical hole down to several hundred feet above the target reservoir, which is generally 2,000 to 9,000 feet below the surface, then turning the drill bit through an arc until it is drilling essentially horizontally. Hydraulic fracturing fluid is then injected under controlled high pressure to fracture, or disrupt, the rock while a proppant (typically quartz sand grains) carried in the fluid props open the fracture after the fluid pressure is released. The propped fracture provides the permeability necessary for the gas to flow from the formation into the well.

A proppant is a material that will keep an induced hydraulic fracture open, during or following a fracturing treatment, and is used to aid in the extraction of oil and gas from reservoir rocks. It is mainly used in the hydraulic fracturing process to increase the productivity of natural gas and oil wells. There are currently three types of proppant: quartz sand, resin-coated sand, and ceramic sand, which is the strongest.

Typical high-pressure, high-volume hydraulic fracturing fluids (HVHFFs) contain different chemicals of various types, manufacture, and concentration, including water, sand (a "proppant"), and low concentrations of chemical additives, generally consisting of friction reducers, biocides to prevent bacterial development, and scale inhibitors. Despite the routine presence of similar, or identical, chemicals in much higher concentrations in many American foodstuffs, medications, cosmetics, and household cleaners, much has been published about potential environmental and human-health impact from the additive components of the HVHFFs. However, most of these published reports lack critical analyses and discussions of dose-response relationships, which are crucial to understanding toxicity arguments.

The paper upon which this brochure is based is an exhaustive inquiry and investigation seeking evidence of adverse public health effects from fracking: No such evidence was found, and all available data suggest the process is completely safe in terms of public health. There are zero confirmable cases of high-volume hydrofracturing-related adverse human-health impact in local residents. This is not to say that the cited lack of current, documented evidence of adverse human-health effects should be construed as a definitive, broad-based denial of such. Ongoing study of longer-term health-related outcomes is required. ■

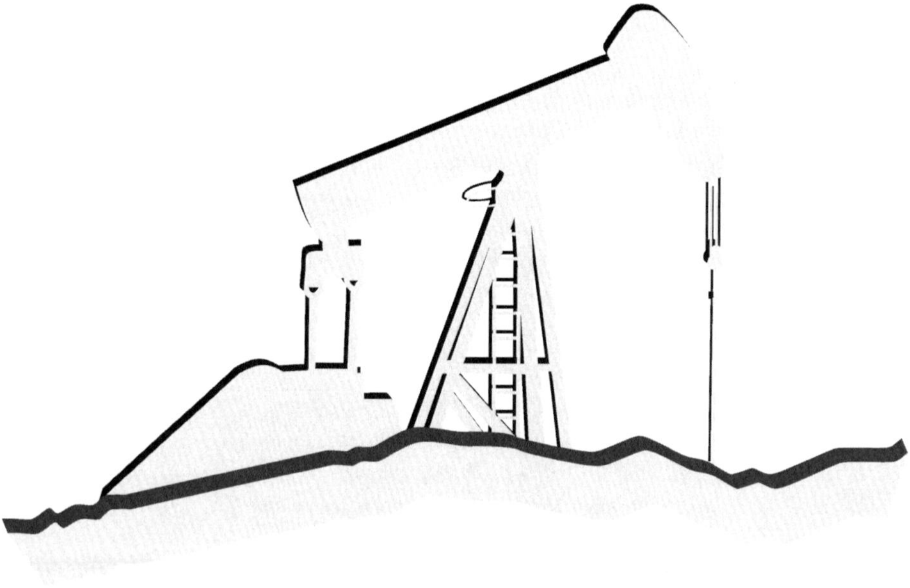

1 INTRODUCTION

Increased awareness about using a highly technical process called hydraulic fracturing to recover natural gas trapped deep within shale deposits has created questions about related human-health and environmental impacts. Associated arguments, both pro and con, have often been subjective, emotional, and unscientific. This paper is aimed at a systematic, objective review of documented types and rates of hydrofracturing-fluid- and chemical-related incidents affecting human health, to date, in the region of the Marcellus Shale Play (**see Map, MCOR, page 11**).

Unconventional gas, consisting primarily of shale gas and tight gas, is playing an increasingly important role America's energy future mainly because technological innovations now are enabling the development and exploitation of underground reserves once considered unrecoverable. Domestic sources of shale gas long have been known to exist.

"Tight gas" *refers to natural gas reservoirs locked in highly impermeable, hard shale. It can also be trapped in sandstone or limestone formations that are similarly impermeable/nonporous.* ***"Tight shale"*** *is impermeable shale rock.* ***"Shale play"*** *is a geographic area that has been deemed suitable for oil and/or gas exploration due to favorable geo-seismic survey findings or productive results from other wells in the same area or region. Such an area comes into play when it is confirmed that there is in fact an economically-rewarding quantity of gas or oil to be developed.* ***"Unconventional (natural) gas"*** *is essentially the same as conventional gas; the term simply refers to the methods that are used, as well as the types of rock from which the oil and natural gas are produced. It refers to natural gas found in low-permeability shale rock; natural gas locked in fine-grained, organic-rich rock (shale gas); and natural gas contained in coal.*

The earliest recorded natural gas discoveries were made by seventeenth-century French explorers and missionaries in the New World. Approximately two centuries later, in 1821, the very first well intended specifically to produce natural gas in the United States was dug near the town of Fredonia in Chautauqua County, New York.

Excavated by hand to a depth of 27 feet, the well supplied gas to the town for illumination (Roen, 1993). It marked the first commercial natural gas production in the United States (Curtis, 2002).

Drilling for natural gas commenced in Pennsylvania in the 1850s and extended into Ohio a decade later (Janssens and de Witt, 1976). Gas subsequently was found in shales in the western Kentucky part of the Illinois Basin in 1863 (Curtis, 2002). By the 1920s, drilling for shale gas had progressed into West Virginia, Kentucky, and Indiana (Curtis, 2002), and by 1926 the Devonian shale-gas fields of eastern Kentucky and West Virginia comprised the largest known natural gas occurrences in the world (Roen, 1993).

Over the decades, as new shale-gas discoveries were made, it became apparent that the only economic use of the black shale was as a source of gas. By the mid-1930s, it was established that gas production from black shale depended on naturally occurring cracks, or fractures, in the rock. Without the fractures, the gas could not escape to the surface. Downhole explosive techniques were introduced to enhance existing fractures in the shale and also to create new ones. While the techniques worked, the results weren't entirely satisfactory, and by the 1950s underground explosives began to be replaced with a new process known as "hydrafrac," in which liquids and proppants were pumped under high pressure into selective shale zones for fracture enhancement. The technique was quite successful, and modified versions are still in use (Roen, 1993). ■

2 U.S. SHALE GAS PRODUCTION

The U.S. Energy Information Administration's (EIA) Annual Energy Outlook 2013 projects U.S. natural gas production to increase from 23.0 trillion cubic feet in 2011 to 33.1 trillion cubic feet in 2040, a 44 percent increase. Almost all of the increase in domestic natural gas output is due to projected growth in shale gas production. Half of all U.S. natural gas production is expected to come from shale by the year 2040. The U.S. produced 7.8 trillion cubic feet (Tcf) of shale gas in 2011 compared with just 0.52 Tcf in 2003, when shale accounted for only 2.7 percent of total U.S. gas output. In 2011, shale's share of total natural gas production was 34.1 percent. EIA's Annual Energy Outlook 2013 projects shale gas output will rise to 12.84 Tcf by 2025, or 44.9 percent of all domestic gas production, and to 16.70 Tcf by 2040, representing 50.4 percent of total U.S. natural gas output (EIA, AEO2013).

The present-day revolution in shale gas took place virtually overnight. In the five years from 2004 to 2009, U.S. shale-gas production quadrupled from 2 billion cubic feet per day (BCFD) to more than 8 BCFD (Stevens and Kuuskraa, 2009). It began with the Barnett Shale in North Texas and was followed by the development of the Fayetteville Shale in Arkansas, the Woodford Shale in Oklahoma, the Haynesville/Bossier Formations in Louisiana and Texas, the Marcellus Shale in the Appalachian Basin, and the Eagle Ford in Texas. Together with the Bakken shale in North Dakota, these are the most active producing gas shales to date (USGS 2013). ■

NATURAL GAS PRODUCTION BY SOURCE, 1990–2040 (TRILLION CUBIC FEET)

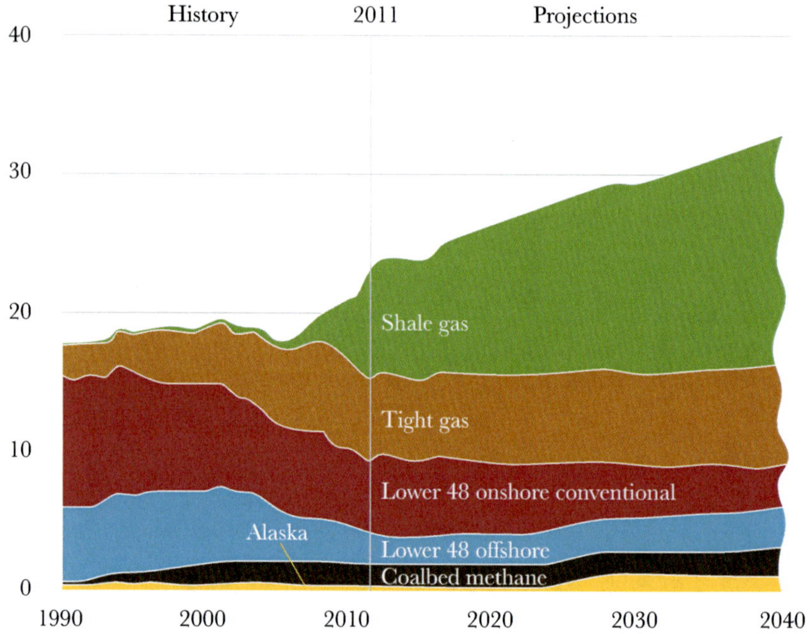

Source: EIA, AEO2013

3 THE MARCELLUS SHALE

Shales are present in sedimentary basins across North America, including the lower 48 states and Alaska. These basins originally were bodies of water where sediments and organic material were deposited over long periods of time millions of years ago. The Devonian-aged shales of the Appalachian, Illinois, and Michigan basins, for example, were deposited approximately 385 million years ago. In comparison, the Barnett and Fayetteville shales were deposited during the late Mississippian Period (about 325 million years ago) and the Haynesville-Bossier shale during the Jurassic period (approximately 150 million years ago). If the volume of organic material contained within the shale is significant, it can serve as a source rock for oil and gas as the buried material is subjected to high heat and pressure over millions of years.

*The term **"conventional gas"** describes natural gas accumulations found in high permeability rock formations, typically sandstones or carbonates, where the hydrocarbons have migrated from finer grained source rocks like shales. These natural gas accumulations include some sort of trapping mechanism that prevents the gas from migrating further and results in a high concentration of gas within the reservoir. "Unconventional gas," in comparison, refers to natural gas found in the shale source rocks themselves (i.e., shale gas), in very low permeability sandstones (i.e., tight gas), or in coal seams (i.e., coalbed methane). In conventional oil and gas reservoirs, the hydrocarbons are located within interconnected pore spaces that allow flow to the wellbore. This "interconnectedness" (or permeability) is severely limited in shale reservoirs (NETL, 2013).*

This study focuses on the Devonian Marcellus Formation, or Marcellus Shale, a sedimentary rock formation deposited over 350 million years ago in a shallow inland sea located in the eastern United States where the Appalachian Mountains now stand (de Witt and others, 1993). The formation gets its name from an outcropping found near Marcellus, New York during a geological survey in 1839 (Penn State Extension, 2014). The Marcellus Shale covers an area of more than 100,000 square miles. Nine states overlie the shale deposit: Kentucky, Maryland, New Jersey, New York, Ohio, Pennsylvania, Tennessee, Virginia, and West Virginia. The organic-rich, gas-producing layers of the Marcellus Shale range from less than 5 feet thick to more than 250 feet thick, with the approximate depth to the base ranging from about 2,000 feet to 9,000 feet below ground surface. At greater depths, the overlying rocks cause greater pressure in the Marcellus formation which can result in higher production rates if properly stimulated. In general, with greater depth, the natural gas contains higher proportions of methane and less propane, butane, and ethane (Penn State MCOR, 2014).

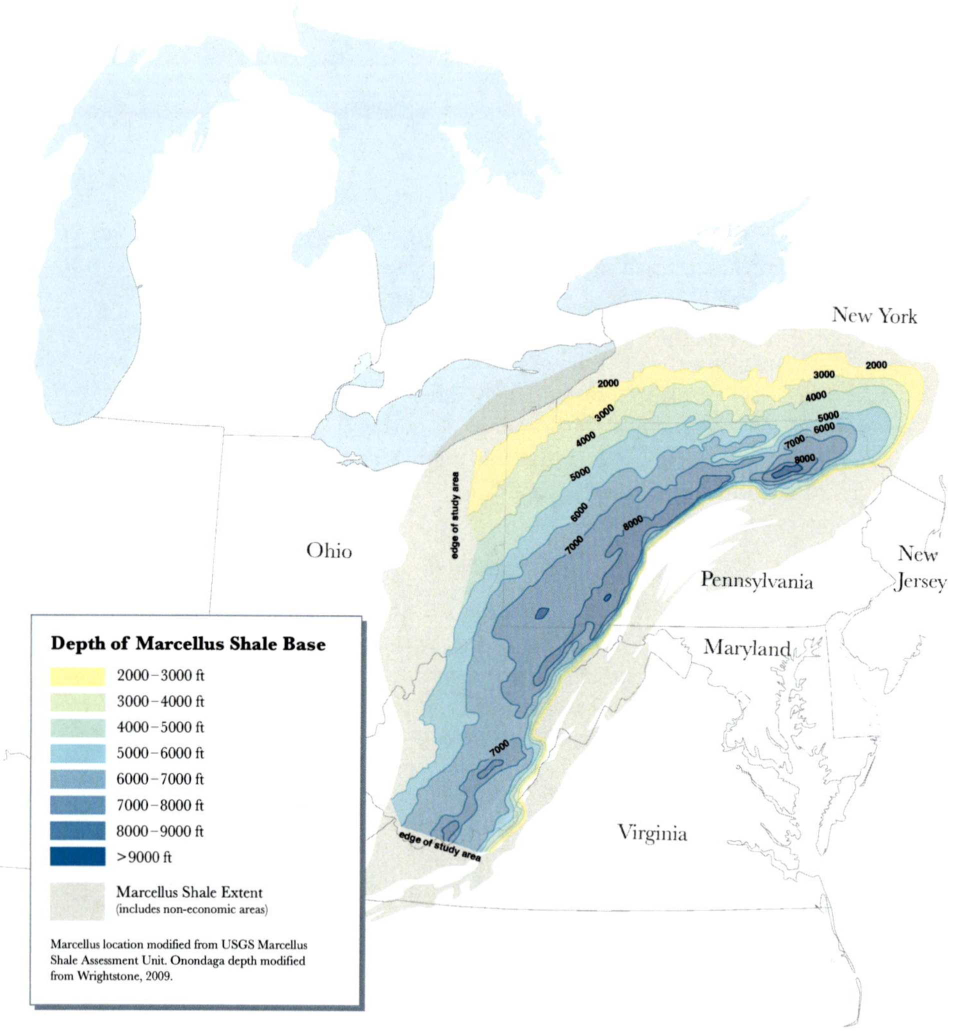

Source: Penn State MCOR, 2014

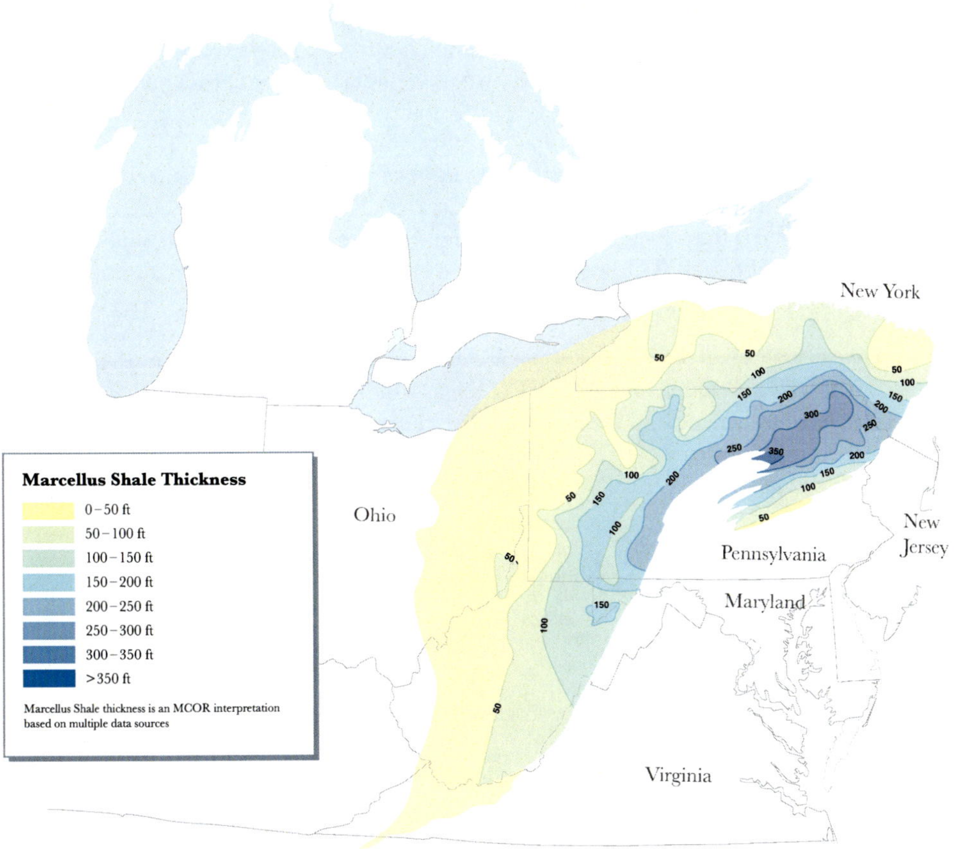

Source: Penn State MCOR, 2014

The Marcellus Shale contains about 84 Tcf of undiscovered, technically recoverable natural gas and 3.4 billion barrels of undiscovered, technically recoverable natural gas liquids, according to an assessment by the U. S. Geological Survey (USGS). The estimates are significantly larger than the prior USGS assessment of the Marcellus Shale in the Appalachian Basin in 2002. The increase in undiscovered, technically recoverable resource is due to new geologic information and engineering data, as technological developments in producing unconventional resources have been significant in the last decade.

New developments in drilling technology, along with higher wellhead prices, have made the Marcellus Shale an important natural gas resource (Soeder and Kappel, 2009). The Marcellus is characterized as a "tight" shale, with vertical fractures (or "joints") that are few and naturally occurring. This necessitates the application of horizontal, subsurface drilling techniques, with engineering procedures that invoke subsequent, high-pressure, high-volume hydraulic fracturing (HVHF) and related techniques in order to make gas recovery both voluminous and financially feasible. Tight shales require fracturing because, although they are very porous, those pores are not interconnected and are also known as "not permeable" because of this. The fracturing process creates an artificial permeability by breaking these rocks apart and, therefore, allowing natural gas to flow up, through the well. The lack of natural vertical joints is actually a benefit from a safety perspective in that vertical fractures would facilitate gas migration upward toward the surface. The production of commercial quantities of gas from this shale requires large volumes of water to drill and hydraulically fracture the rock. This water must be recovered from the well and disposed of before the gas can flow (Soeder and Kappel, 2009).

The geologic cross section (below) depicts the extent and depth of the Marcellus Shale near Clearfield, Pennsylvania. Found as deep as 9,000 feet below the ground surface in northeastern and central Pennsylvania, the Marcellus Formation generally becomes shallower at depths of 2,000 feet toward northwest Pennsylvania. The Marcellus Shale underlies nearly 75 percent of Pennsylvania (Penn State MCOR, 2014). ■

GENERALIZED GEOLOGIC CROSS SECTION SHOWING MARCELLUS SHALE IN WESTERN PENNSYLVANIA

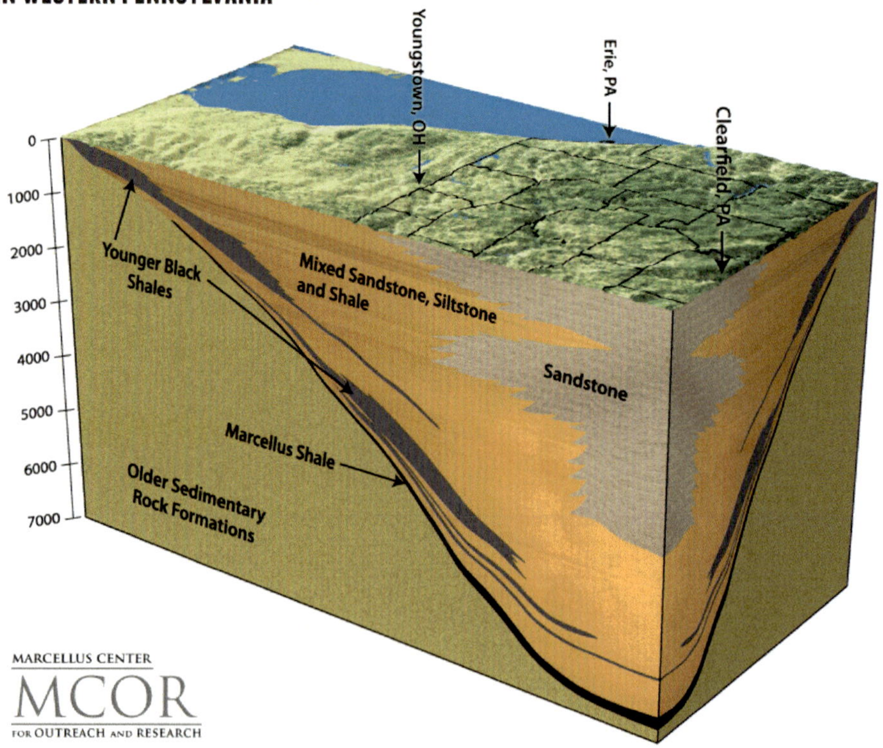

MARCELLUS CENTER MCOR FOR OUTREACH AND RESEARCH

Source: Penn State MCOR, 2014

4 RECOVERY TECHNOLOGIES

The low natural permeability of shale has been the limiting factor in the exploitation of shale gas (Denney, 2009), but the advent of horizontal drilling and hydraulic fracturing have facilitated the expansion of modern shale-gas development (USGS 2013). Although the first horizontal well was drilled in Texas in 1929, it was not until the 1980s that the technology was improved enough to become a standard industry practice. The technology involves drilling a vertical hole to several hundred feet above the target reservoir, then directing the drill bit through an arc until it is drilling essentially horizontally (Harper, 2008). The advantages of horizontal wells include increases in the amount of reservoir penetrated from possibly hundreds of feet to over 5,000 feet, and increases in the number of vertical or sub-vertical fractures intersected (Stevens and Kuuskraa, 2009, USGS 2013).

A horizontal well (as depicted on page 18) starts with vertical drilling followed by horizontal drilling. Vertical drilling in the Marcellus Shale ranges from 5,000 feet to 9,000 feet below ground, depending on the depth and thickness of the gas reservoir. When the Marcellus Shale is reached, the drill is turned, and horizontal drilling occurs for an additional 3,000 feet to 10,000 feet or more. At various depths, multiple lengths of steel casing are cemented in place to protect surface water, groundwater, or water supply wells from the potential migration of natural gas in the drilled well. These casings also prevent hydrofracking fluids and deep brine water from leaking and adversely impacting water resources (Penn State MCOR, 2014).

The first step in the well completion process involves perforating the well casing in the horizontal portion of the well. A string of shaped explosive charges is detonated electrically in the casing across from the zone to be hydraulically fractured, perforating the casing and cement. Hydraulic fracturing fluid is then injected under controlled high pressure to part the rock while a proppant (typically quartz sand grains) carried in the fluid props open the fracture after the fluid pressure is released and the fracture begins to close. The propped fracture provides the permeability necessary for the gas to flow from the formation into the well. As many as 25 or more such treatments may be pumped within a single wellbore. Hydraulic fracturing of shale gas formations typically

CROSS-SECTION OF TYPICAL HORIZONTAL MARCELLUS WELL

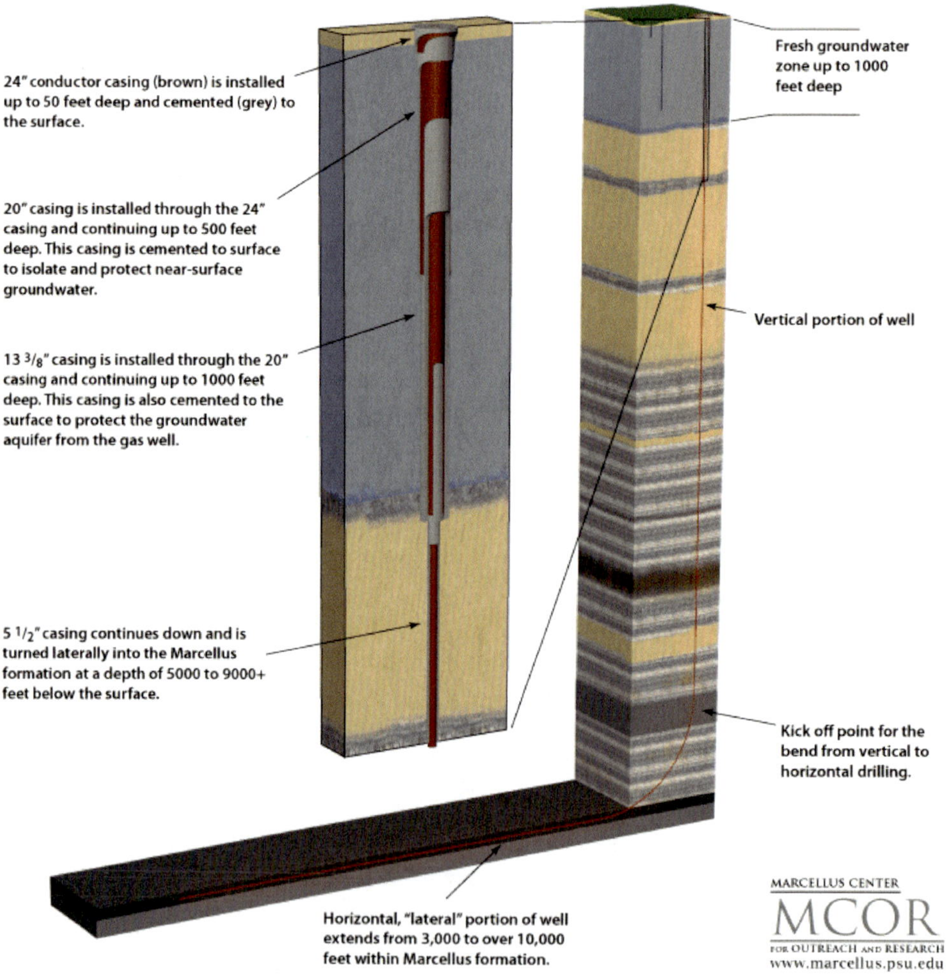

Source: Penn State MCOR, 2014

requires the use of 3 to 6 million gallons of water per well. In the Marcellus, roughly 20 percent to 25 percent of the water injected will come out of the well as "flowback water." Over the life of the well, additional volumes of the water will be produced. Both the flowback water and the produced water must be separated from the gas and hydrocarbon liquids, and either cleaned up and reused or disposed of in deep disposal wells. In some plays in the U.S., more than 90 percent of flowback water is reused in fracturing other wells (NETL, 2013).

Typical high-pressure, high-volume hydraulic fracturing fluids (HVHFFs) contain different chemicals of various types, manufacture, and concentration, including water, sand, biocides, rust/scale inhibitors, "acidizers" (acidifiers), other pH-adjusting agents, breakers, oxygen scavengers, crosslinkers, clay inhibitors, clay stabilizers, gelling agents, surfactants, and others. Some of these formulations remain proprietary; some have been made public. Representative, contributory fractions to the multichemical content of the HVHFFs are seen below in a sample composition, by weight, of fracturing fluid based on data from Marcellus Shale development in Pennsylvania. Between 84 and 90 percent of the fracturing fluid is water; between approximately 8 and 15 percent is proppant; the remainder, typically less than 1 percent consists of chemical additives (NYSDEC 2011). The relatively small amounts of additives generally consist of friction reducers, biocides to prevent bacterial development, and scale inhibitors.

SAMPLE FRACTURING FLUID COMPOSITION (9 ADDITIVES), BY WEIGHT, FROM MARCELLUS SHALE

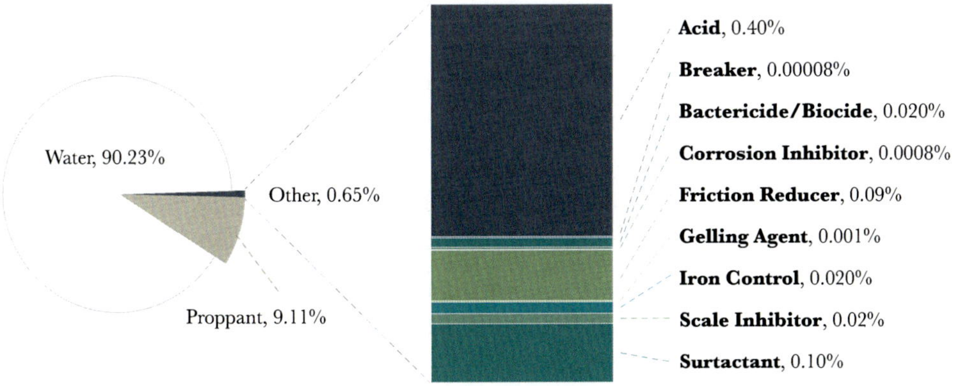

Source: NYSDEC 2011

The number of chemical additives used in a typical fracture treatment depends on the conditions of the specific well being fractured. A typical fracture treatment will use very low concentrations of between 3 and 12 additive chemicals, depending on the characteristics of the water and the shale formation. Each component serves a specific engineering purpose. For example, the predominant fluids currently being used for fracture treatments are water-based fracturing fluids mixed with friction-reducing additives (called slickwater). The addition of friction reducers allows fracturing fluids and proppants to be pumped to the target zone at a higher rate and lower pressure than if water alone were used.

Despite the routine presence of similar, or identical, chemicals in many American foodstuffs, medications, cosmetics, and household cleaners in much higher concentrations, much has been published about potential environmental and human-health impact from the additive components of the HVHFFs. However, most of these published reports are lacking critical analyses and discussions of dose-response relationships so important in communicating scientifically-valid toxicity arguments. The dose makes the poison: the HVHFF chemicals are present in such low concentrations so as not to pose a realistic health concern.

The hydrofracturing process is associated with both natural and engineered barriers to natural-gas flow, leakage, and contamination from the Marcellus wells, including distance/depth, steel and cement/steel well casings, blow-out preventers, pressure sensors, and many complex series of control valves and manifolds. Chemical-transportation controls, specifically, involve appropriately rated vehicles, the routine use of federally mandated vehicle placarding, and controlled volumes of HVHFF chemicals. Well site surface-safety controls require controlled access/security, chemical isolation/protection, and personal protective equipment (PPE) for nearby workers. Surface controls at the wellhead also include pressure-rated plumbing and hardware; pressure and flow sensors/alarms; impermeable surface/ground mats; mixing and injecting controllers; holding/waste ponds; recovering/recycling; and processing of HVHFF chemicals. In the active-drilling Marcellus zones, flowback water is subject to processing/cleanup prior to discharge, and as much as 90 percent of that flowback water is reused at different well sites.

Downhole safety measures concerning HVHFFs also include pressure-rated plumbing and hardware; well casings (typically now triple-steel/cement in the area of groundwater aquifers and the vertical component of the well shafts); blowout preventers; flow/position/pressure monitors and sensors; and simple geologic depth — thousands of feet as a rule. Despite these numerous safeguards, there remains a great deal of public skepticism as to their individual and collective reliabilities and effectiveness in preventing HVHFF contamination of well site surfaces, groundwater, air, and surface water. ■

5 HYDROFRACTURING AND HUMAN HEALTH

The original study upon which this version is based was an observational compendium of objective data, whose goal was to characterize and quantify any and all subsurface, HVHF-related incidents that, to date, have actually adversely affected human health in the distribution of natural-gas drilling and production activities in the Marcellus. This study is restricted to the actual hydrofracturing process itself. It does not cover the surface or subsurface activities of drilling, the building of related roads or pipelines, or the processes of casing a well — all of which are common to drilling of *any* well for *any* purpose. Nor do we address air quality.

Of the three states with active Marcellus HVHF drilling, two of them, namely Ohio and West Virginia, have not experienced any officially documented, adverse human-health events related to that activity, even with hundreds of wells already having been drilled there. Pennsylvania, the state with the highest level of HVHF activity in the Marcellus Shale, with roughly 10,000 wells drilled there from 2008 to date, has experienced roughly 40 related environmental incidents ("spills into navigable waters") in which the U.S. Environmental Protection Agency (US EPA) became involved via its Region 3 office, none of which apparently rose to the level of adverse human-health events. The US EPA has become embroiled in many cases of suspected, Marcellus-related environmental disruption, including the infamous one of alleged, widespread groundwater contamination of domestic wells by migrating methane in Dimock, Pennsylvania (Star Gazette, 2009, Lustgarten, 2009). However, the US EPA closed its investigation, with findings that the level of contamination was below federal safety triggers (Entine, 2013). Similarly, the US EPA has either terminated and/or otherwise significantly revised its investigations into several other allegedly HVHF-related incidents in many other states/shale plays (Entine, 2013).

With respect to the study at hand, the EPA's total tallies on alleged, Marcellus HVHF-related environmental infractions were sourced from the US EPA Region 3's verbal representations of approximately 40 incidents of "spills into navigable waters" that had risen to its level of review. ***None of the 40 incidents, however, rose to the level of documented human-health impact.*** US EPA Region 3 holds purview over several states relevant to this review, including Maryland (no Marcellus drilling), Pennsylvania (roughly 10,000 Marcellus wells), Virginia (no Marcellus drilling), and West Virginia (roughly 1,100 Marcellus wells). As for Ohio, where the remainder of the Marcellus drilling activity is located (with roughly 460 wells), the state falls in US EPA Region 5, in which there was no report of US EPA involvement in any related incident.

The Pennsylvania Department of Environmental Protection (PA DEP), according to press reports, has been actively investigating claims of alleged domestic water-well and surface-spring contamination from HVHF-related drilling. Of 973 complaints, none was determined to be *directly* causally related to HVHF activity. While the presence of methane in domestic water was, in some cases, determined by the PA DEP to be causally related to "contamination of water supplies from oil and gas operations," in other cases the PA DEP found no relationship to "oil and gas operations." There have been sporadic reports of findings of levels of methane in homes near Marcellus drilling activities, but there have been no citations of related explosions or injuries to humans or human health. Moreover, given the recent findings of methane in well water in 15 percent of 66 domestic wells tested by the U.S. Geological Service in the immediately neighboring upstate/Southern Tier area of New York (which directly overlies the Marcellus shale) in the complete absence of related drilling and in the presence of a related drilling ban, the question arises as to whether such findings result from Marcellus drilling or simply from naturally occurring methane migration from underground sources. Those New York wells were more than one mile away from existing or abandoned natural gas wells, and the levels of methane were high enough to warrant monitoring or remediation (Begos, 2013). Therefore the methane in the wells was clearly biogenic, i.e., naturally-occurring. There is no valid, scientific reason to believe that the same phenomenon is not occurring in Pennsylvania. ■

6 CONCLUSIONS

To date, there has been no Marcellus Shale high-volume hydrofracturing activity in Kentucky, Maryland, New Jersey, Tennessee, or Virginia, and, therefore, there has been no related human-health impact. In New York State, which overlies the Marcellus and experienced historical hydrofracturing activity since the 1980s, there is an absence of any officially recorded incidence of HVHF-related human-health impacts from those activities. Likewise, Internet searches failed to produce any objective, traceable data on adverse human-health impacts Furthermore, given the absence of post-ban HVHF-type drilling in New York, one would not logically expect any such impacts. Similarly, Region 2 of the US EPA, which oversees New York, did not provide requested data on any such incidents. It is, once again, likely that there are no responsive documents from those sources and that there is a 0 percent related incidence of HVHF-related, adverse human-health impacts in Region 2, including New York.

The presence of methane in appreciable, if not remedial-level, amounts in 15 percent of 66 domestic water wells tested in southern New York — in spite of the absence of current Marcellus, HVHF-type drilling and at least one mile distance from any existing well — suggests that background levels of methane in that geographic region are not associated with Marcellus, HVHF-type drilling. There may be parallel situations elsewhere in the Marcellus distribution, and those situations should be objectively addressed in terms of their ultimate sources. Resultant knowledge should be integrated into future regulations regarding HVHF-sourced drilling and production in the Marcellus.

Where there is current, Marcellus-related HVHF activity in Ohio, Pennsylvania, and West Virginia and where roughly 11,560 total Marcellus wells have been drilled, there is a collective incidence of state-level environmental cases or claims of roughly 10 percent in Pennsylvania and 0 percent in both Ohio and West Virginia. In addition, Regions 3 and 5 of the US EPA have each apparently experienced a 0 percent incidence of adverse human-health impact from the Marcellus HVHF activities, reported by them as "no data responsive." While there have been numerous cases of adverse environmental impact in Pennsylvania, apparently from surface activities, there has been a 0 percent incidence of associated documented, adverse human-health impact.

The current incidence of acute, adverse human-health impact from the hydrofracturing process itself within the active Marcellus zones appears to be 0 percent, according to the figures and to information made available by government agencies and reliable secondary sources. These data, in turn, suggest that, to date, actual HVHF within the active Marcellus zones has been, in very simple terms, 100 percent safe with respect to acute, adverse, human-health impacts. This is not to say that the cited lack of current, documented evidence of adverse human-health effects from HVHF in the Marcellus should be construed as a definitive, broad-based denial of such future possible discoveries, i.e. of adverse health effects related to proximity to HVHF activities. Authorities should continue to look for any HVHF-related, adverse human-health effects on residents in close, intermediate, and relatively distant proximities to HVHF activities/areas in the Marcellus. Such medical surveillance is a common-sense matter and would provide the "video" perspective in this matter, which may prove superior to the present "snapshot" one. A related database should be established, tracking all such claims and findings, by type, location, geology, and definitive etiology (where possible). Standardized, published, traceable standards and methodologies for such causation determinations should be established and consistently applied if any sense is to be made, or conclusions drawn, from such a database. ■

7 REFERENCES

Begos, K., Study finds methane in 15 percent of upstate N.Y. wells, Associated Press in Star Gazette (Elmira, NY), Dec 17, 2013 http://www.stargazette.com/viewart/20131217/NEWS01/312170062/Study-finds-methane-15-percent-upstate-N-Y-wells.

Coleman, J.L., Milici, R.C., Cook, T.A., Charpentier, R.R., Kirschbaum, Mark, Klett, T.R., Pollastro, R.M., and Schenk, C.J., 2011, Assessment of undiscovered oil and gas resources of the Devonian Marcellus Shale of the Appalachian Basin Province, 2011: U.S. Geological Survey Fact Sheet 2011–3092, 2 p., available at http://pubs.usgs.gov/fs/2011/3092/.

Curtis, J.B., 2002, Fractured shale–gas systems: American Association of Petroleum Geologists Bulletin, v. 86, no. 11, p. 1921–1938. Accessed on May 12, 2010 at http://search.datapages.com/data/bulletns/2002/11nov/1921/images/02_1921.pdf.

Davis, R., Jr. 1992, "Depositional Systems: An Introduction to Sedimentology and Stratigraphy," Prentice Hall, 2nd Edition, 1992 in National Energy Technology Laboratory, 2013, Modern shale gas development in the United States: an update, Strategic Center for Natural Gas and Oil, U.S. Department of Energy, September 2013, http://www.netl.doe.gov/File%20Library/Research/Oil-Gas/shale-gas-primer-update-2013.pdf.

de Witt, Wallace, Jr., Roen, J.B., and Wallace, L.G., 1993, Stratigraphy of Devonian black shales and associated rocks in the Appalachian basin, in Roen, J.B., and Kepferle, R.C., eds., Petroleum geology of the Devonian and Mississippian black shale of eastern North America: U.S. Geological Survey Bulletin 1909–B, p. B1–B57 http://pubs.er.usgs.gov/publication/b1909.

Entine, J., Will Washington politics kill the U.S. energy revival and shale gas revolution? Forbes, Aug. 22, 2013, http://www.forbes.com/sites/jonentine/2013/08/22/will-washington-politics-kill-the-us-energy-revival-and-shale-gas-revolution/2/.

FracFocus, Chemical use in hydraulic fracturing, 2014, http://fracfocus.org/water-protection/drilling-usage.

Harper, J.A., 2008, The Marcellus Shale—An old "new" gas reservoir in Pennsylvania: Pennsylvania Geology, v. 38, no. 1. in U.S. Geological Survey (USGS) National Assessment of Oil and Gas Resources Team, and Biewick, L.R.H., compiler, 2013, Map of assessed shale gas in the United States, 2012: U.S. Geological Survey Digital Data Series 69–Z, 16 p., 1 pl., GIS data package, http://pubs.usgs.gov/dds/dds-069/dds-069-z/.

Hill, D.G., Curtis, J.B., and Lillis, P.G., 2008, Update on North America shale-gas exploration and development, in Hill, D.G., Lillis, P.G., and Curtis, J.B., eds., 2008, Gas shale in the Rocky Mountains and beyond, 2008 Guidebook: Rocky Mountain Association of Geologists, Denver, Colo. in U.S. Geological Survey (USGS) National Assessment of Oil and Gas Resources Team, and Biewick, L.R.H., compiler, 2013, Map of assessed shale gas in the United States, 2012: U.S. Geological Survey Digital Data Series 69–Z, 16 p., 1 pl., GIS data package, http://pubs.usgs.gov/dds/dds-069/dds-069-z/.

Janssens, Adriaan, and de Witt, Wallace, Jr., 1976, Potential natural gas resources in the Devonian shales of Ohio: Geological Note no. 3. State of Ohio, Department of Natural Resources, Division of Geological Survey, Columbus, Ohio, 12 p. in U.S. Geological Survey (USGS) National Assessment of Oil and Gas Resources Team, and Biewick, L.R.H., compiler, 2013, Map of assessed shale gas in the United States, 2012: U.S. Geological Survey Digital Data Series 69–Z, 16 p., 1 pl., GIS data package, http://pubs.usgs.gov/dds/dds-069/dds-069-z/.

Lustgarten, A., Does natural gas drilling make water burn? Scientific American, Apr 27, 2009, http://www.scientificamerican.com/article/natural-gas-make-water-burn/

National Energy Technology Laboratory, 2013, Modern shale gas development in the United States: an update, Strategic Center for Natural Gas and Oil, U.S. Department of Energy, September 2013, http://www.netl.doe.gov/File%20Library/Research/Oil-Gas/shale-gas-primer-update-2013.pdf.

New York State Department of Environmental Conservation, Revised Draft, Supplemental Generic Environmental Impact Statement (SGEIS) on the oil, gas and solution mining regulatory program, Sec. 5 Natural gas development activities and high-volume hydraulic fracturing, (September 2011) http://www.dec.ny.gov/energy/75370.html.

Penn State Extension, 2014, Devonian Marcellus Formation Maps, College of Agricultural Sciences, Penn State http://extension.psu.edu/natural-resources/natural-gas/maps/devonian.

Penn State Marcellus Center for Outreach and Research, MCOR, Penn State, 2014 http://www.marcellus.psu.edu/resources/maps.php.

Roen, J.B., 1993, Introductory review—Devonian and Mississippian black shale, eastern North America, in Roen, J.B., and Kepferle, R.C., eds., Petroleum Geology of the Devonian and Mississippian black shale of eastern North America: U.S. Geological Survey Bulletin 1909, p. A1–A8. Available at http://pubs.usgs.gov/bul/1909/report.pdf.

Soeder, D.J., and Kappel, W.M., 2009, Water resources and natural gas production from the Marcellus Shale: U.S. Geological Survey Fact Sheet 2009–3032, 6 p. http://pubs.usgs.gov/fs/2009/3032/.

Star Gazette (Elmira, NY), Pa. orders a halt to Cabot gas drilling in Dimock, Sept. 25, 2009, http://www.stargazette.com/article/20090925/NEWS01/90925025/1117/news/Pa.+orders+a+halt+to+Cabot+gas+drilling+in+Dimock.

Stevens, S. and Kuuskraa, V., 2009, Special Report: Gas Shale 1—Seven plays dominate North America activity: Oil & Gas Journal, September 28, 2009, p. 39–49. Accessed on July 9, 2012 at http://www.ogj.com/articles/print/volume-107/issue-36/Drilling___Production/special-report-gas-shale-1-seven-plays-dominate-north-america-activity.html.

U.S. Energy Information Administration (EIA), The Annual Energy Outlook 2013 (AEO2013), Office of Integrated and International Energy Analysis, U.S. Department of Energy, Washington, DC, April 2013, available at http://www.eia.gov/forecasts/aeo.

U.S. Geological Survey (USGS) National Assessment of Oil and Gas Resources Team, and Biewick, L.R.H., compiler, 2013, Map of assessed shale gas in the United States, 2012: U.S. Geological Survey Digital Data Series 69–Z, 16 p., 1 pl., GIS data package, http://pubs.usgs.gov/dds/dds-069/dds-069-z/.

Wrightstone, Gregory, 2009, Marcellus Shale—Geologic controls on production, adapted from extended abstract prepared for oral presentation at American Association of Petroleum Geologists Annual Convention, Denver, Colo., June 7–10, 2009 in U.S. Geological Survey (USGS) National Assessment of Oil and Gas Resources Team, and Biewick, L.R.H., compiler, 2013, Map of assessed shale gas in the United States, 2012: U.S. Geological Survey Digital Data Series 69–Z, 16 p., 1 pl., GIS data package, http://pubs.usgs.gov/dds/dds-069/dds-069-z/.

BOARD OF SCIENTIFIC AND POLICY ADVISORS

BOARD OF SCIENTIFIC AND POLICY ADVISORS (CONTINUED)

BOARD OF SCIENTIFIC AND POLICY ADVISORS (CONTINUED)

BOARD OF SCIENTIFIC AND POLICY ADVISORS (CONTINUED)

BOARD OF SCIENTIFIC AND POLICY ADVISORS (CONTINUED)

The opinions expressed in ACSH publications do not necessarily represent the views of all members of the ACSH Board of Trustees, Founders Circle and Board of Scientific and Policy Advisors, who all serve without compensation.

Made in United States
Orlando, FL
07 November 2026

90337522R00024